Meal Prepping Cookbook for Weight Loss

The Ultimate Beginners Guide to Meal Prep Recipes to Make Ahead of Time - Quick & Easy Packable Breakfasts, Grab & Go Lunches, Fat Burning Dinners Meal Plans

By Abigail Murphy

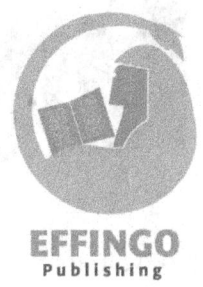

For more great books, visit:

EffingoPublishing.com

Download another book for Free

We want to thank you for purchasing this book and offer you another book (just as long and valuable as this book), "To be mentioned later," completely free.

Visit the link below to signup and receive it:

www.effingopublishing.com/gift

In this book, we will break down the most common health & fitness mistakes, you are probably committing right now, and will reveal how you can quickly get in the best shape of your life!

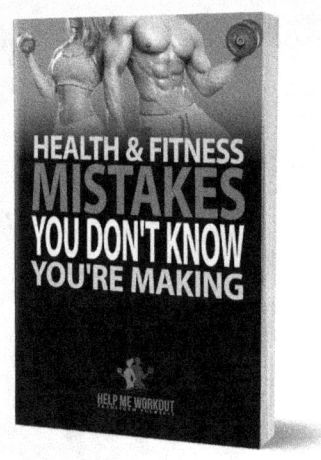

In addition to this valuable gift, you will also have an opportunity to get our new books for free, enter giveaways, and receive other useful emails from us. Again, visit the link to sign up:

www.effingopublishing.com/gift

TABLE OF CONTENT

Introduction 8

"Long Term Meal" 9

"Short Term Meal" 10

Chapter 1: Food That Matters- Meal Prepping Principles 12

Make it Simple 12

Cook in Batches 13

Cook different with same recipes 13

Keep Ingredients Fresh 13

Make a shopping list 14

Food Safety 14

Chapter 02: Easy & Healthy Breakfast to Lose Weight 15

Smoked Salmon Breakfast Flatbread 15

Scrambled Tofu Breakfast Burrito (30 minutes) 18

Spicy Breakfast Fajitas with Eggs and Guacamole..... 21

Banana and Chocolate Chip Baked Oatmeal Cups..... 24

"Chocolate Chia Overnight Oats" 26

Oatmeal Blueberry Yogurt Pancakes 28

Protein-Packed Breakfast Acron Squash 30

Chapter 03: Best Quick & Easy Recipes to Lose Weight (Lunch) 48

Indian Shrimp Curry 48

Roast beef and Horse Radish 51

Tuna Avocado Sandwich 52

Pepper and Onion Wraps 53

Salmon & Avocado Salad with Lemon Dressing 55

Lemon Pepper Salmon Caesar Salad 57

Avocado & Grape Salad with Walnuts 60

Skinny Burrito in a jar 62

Protein Cobb Salad with Quinoa 63

Sprouts, Veggies, and Cheese Wrap 65

Creamy Sweet Potato and Pear Soup 67

Lentil & Kale Soup 69

Avocado Chicken Wrap 71

Japanese Tuna Salad 74

Asian Chicken & Veggie Lettuce Wraps 75

Chapter 04: Deliciously Healthy Dinner Recipes for Weight Loss 78

Rosemary Citrus One Pan Baked Salmon 78

Mushroom and Black Bean Smothered Burritos 81

Arroz Con Pollo, Lightened Up. 84

Healthy Greek Chicken and Farro Salad 87

Instant Pot Beef and Barley Stew 89

Coconut-Lime Marinated Shrimp and Noodles 91

Grilled Watermelon + Steak Salad 94

Smashed Pea and Ricotta Pappardelle 96

Grilled Chicken with Smoky Corn Salad 98

White Beans and Tuna Salad with Basil Vinaigrette..100

Rhubarb and Citrus Salad (Black Pepper Vinaigrette) 102

Pot Sticker Stir-Fry 104

Grilled Basil Chicken and Zucchini 106

Chicago-Style Chicken Dogs 108

Steak and Rye Panzanella 110

Cheesy Tex-Mex Stuffed Chicken 113

Chapter 05: Appetizing Snacks For Weight Loss 115

Avocado Fries with Lime Dipping Sauce 115

Mango-Raspberry Fruit Roll-ups 118

Double Chocolate Paleo Banana Bread 120

Air Fryer Tostones (twice air-fried plantains) 123

Delicious Carrot Cake Cookies (prepared with coconut oil & dairy-free!) 125

No-Bake Superfood Brownie Energy Bars 128

Homemade Chunky Healthy Granola Recipe (vegan & gluten-free!) 131

Vegetarian Plantain & Black Bean Taco Cups 134

Green Goddess Hummus 137

Crispy Baked Sweet Potato Fries 141

Creamy Peach & Honey Popsicles 144

Protein Cookie Dough 146

Almond Joy Protein Balls 149

Baked Kale Chips 151

Chocolate Covered Banana Pops 153

Vitamin c boosting tropical green Smoothie 155

Fruit salad with citrus-mint dressing 157

Conclusion **159**

Final Words **160**

About the Co-Authors **161**

Introduction

Are you looking for a delicious & healthy meal prepping guide book for weight loss? Are you worried about losing weight healthy and quickly?

If yes, you are in the right place

We all understand that consuming healthy food is challenging, and cooking it every day is even tougher. Meal prepping has earned great popularity because it acknowledges both the issues at once. By preparing healthy meals in a large quantity in one setting. You can have delicious and nutritious meals throughout the week without having to worry about wasting time in cooking and cleaning every day.

With this book you will get:

1. Food That Matters- Meal Prepping Principles
2. Easy & Healthy Breakfast to Lose Weight
3. Best Quick & Easy Recipes to Lose Weight (Lunch)
4. Deliciously Healthy Dinner Recipes for Weight Los
5. Tasty Snacks for Weight Loss

Also, before you get started, I recommend you [joining our email newsletter](#) to receive updates on any upcoming new book releases or promotions. You can sign-up for free, and as a bonus, you will receive a gift. I wish you all the best for buying this book "Meal Prepping Cookbook for Weight Loss," I am sure this book will help you manage your relationships.

Meal Prepping can be defined as the daily routine in which you create a preset menu for yourself, and prepare meals when you are running short of time.

It means preparing meals before time, pack them & have them ready when you need them. Meal Prepping has been classified into two categories

"Long Term Meal"

In this category, you can prepare meals for three or more days in advance. Many people organize themselves in such a way that they purchase all the ingredients they need, prepare, and cook everything in the evening. After this, they store the food in "glasses boxes, plastic bags, or other containers. By doing this way, they have their food ready to take with them. This meal-type can take much time and effort, but considering the limited time available, it is worthy of cooking for around 03 to 07 days ahead of time and preparing them in advance.

"Short Term Meal"

In this category, you can prepare meals for a maximum of two days in advance. Many people organize themselves in such a way that they won't have to cook anything when they wake up. They arrange everything in advance, and by the time they wake up, they just need to turn the toaster, and everything is ready. Some people have this habit of marinating meats a day before they need it, to save time. So, these were the categories of Meal preparation.

It ultimately depends on the type of person you are. Some people cook only dinners, whereas some people combine both categories to save time.

So, in this book, we will tell you how to create an effective yet time-saving meal plan. The book consists of delicious recipes, and it will also help you lose weight and enjoy yourself at the same time.

Once again, to join our free email newsletter and to receive a free copy of this valuable book, please visit the link and signup now: www.effingopublishing.com/gift.

Chapter 1: Food That Matters- Meal Prepping Principles

When you are preparing a meal plan, always remember to aim for a healthy lifestyle. Maintaining a healthy lifestyle will keep you energized and focused. Meal preparation is quite easy, and generally, people think it's a difficult job, once you have adopted this habit of meal prep, you will find it a lot easier than before.

Few things that you must consider before Meal Prepare

Make it Simple

It can be difficult if you are doing it for the first time. That's why we recommend you keep things simple and easy. You gain nothing by complicating things. The book consists of recipes that are quite simple to make. We will also offer different recipes for smoothies that you use as a substitute for quick meals. Start with the basics, including beef or chicken. Once you become an expert, you can make your quick recipes and add them to your diet plan.

Cook in Batches

Cooking in batches means to cook a sufficient amount of recipes in one attempt. That means to make around 10 to 12 portions at one time and freezing the rest for the later in a week. It might appear challenging, but in doing so, you are saving time for the rest of your week. So, at times when you don't feel like cooking, just open your fridge and heat the previously prepared food.

Cook different with same recipes

You can always have the option of using the same ingredients and make different dishes with them. By doing so, you won't have to buy anything new, and you can also try a different recipe using the same ingredients

Keep Ingredients Fresh

Keeping vegetables and fruits fresh can be the most challenging thing as they are quickly perishable. Just because of meal prepping things, you shouldn't let loose all the beneficial nutrients from the food. Try to buy food and use them as early as possible. It will help you to maintain a healthy lifestyle.

MAKE A SHOPPING LIST

In such a busy life. Sometimes, maintaining track of everything becomes the most difficult thing. We would recommend keeping a tiny notebook with yourself. The reason for keeping a notebook is because you can note down all the meal plans that you want to create for the week.

FOOD SAFETY

Food safety is an essential principle of all. If you cannot save your food from spoiling, then meal prepping is not for you. Food containers are available in the stores that will help to reduce the air exposure of your meal. Look for the best food containers and buy them in advance.

Chapter 02: Easy & Healthy Breakfast to Lose Weight

Smoked Salmon Breakfast Flatbread

Ingredients:

- 1 cup of "5 oz." white whole wheat flour
- 1 and a half teaspoons of baking powder
- Half teaspoon of kosher salt
- 1 cup of non-fat Greek yogurt, drained if there's any liquid
- Bagel Seasoning
- Half red onion, skinned and sliced into thin strips
- 1 tablespoon of extra virgin olive oil
- 2 ounces 1/2 cup of fat cream cheese
- 1 beefsteak tomato, thinly sliced
- 4 ounces of smoked salmon or nova lox
- 2 tablespoons of capers, drained
- fresh dill, for garnishing

- For gluten-free, I would suggest Cup 4 Cup of flour.

Preparation:

Preheat the oven to 450F.

In a medium dish, mix the flour, baking powder, and salt and beat well.

Put the yogurt and combine with a fork until its combined,

Slightly dust flour on a surface and remove dough from the dish, rub the dough a few times until dough is tacky, but not sticky, around 20 turns (it should not leave the dough on your hand when you pull away).

Divide into 04 balls equally about 3-3/8 oz each.

Drizzle a surface and rolling pin with a little flour roll the dough out into thin ovals 7 to 8 inches in diameter and place on the baking sheet.

Brush the dough with olive oil. Drizzle everything bagel seasoning in a 1-inch border around the edge.

Mix half of the red onion with olive oil, Spread the onion in the center of each.

Take it to the oven and bake for about 10 to 14 minutes, until the crust is golden and crisp.

Remove from oven and dallop cream cheese and leave the edge clear.

Top with tomatoes, then salmon and in the last with capers and dill.

SCRAMBLED TOFU BREAKFAST BURRITO (30 MINUTES)

For TOFU

- 1 "12-ounce" pack of firm tofu
- 1 teaspoon of oil
- 3 garlic cloves (crushed)
- 1 Tablespoon of hummus
- Half teaspoon of chili powder
- Half teaspoon of cumin
- 1 teaspoon of nutritional yeast
- 1/4 teaspoon of sea salt
- 1 pinch of cayenne pepper
- 1/4 cup crushed parsley

Vegetables

- 5 Small potatoes (sliced into bite-size pieces)
- 1 red bell pepper (medium and thinly sliced)
- 1 teaspoon of oil

- 1 pinch of sea salt

- Half teaspoon of ground cumin

- Half teaspoon of chili powder

- 2 cups of sliced kale

- 3-4 large flour

- 1 avocado (medium ripe, sliced or crushed)

- Cilantro

- Solid red or green salsa or hot sauce

Preparation

Preheat oven to 400 degrees (204 C) and stripe a baking sheet with parchment paper. In the meanwhile, also cover tofu in a clean cloth and put something heavy on top

Put potatoes and red pepper to the baking sheet, sprinkle with oil and spices and mix to combine. Bake for around 15-22 minutes or until it becomes tender and lightly browned. Insert kale in the last 5 minutes of baking to wilt, Mix with the other vegetables to combine flavors.

Meanwhile, heat a large pot on medium heat. Once it's hot, add oil, garlic, and tofu and cook for 7-10 minutes, stirring gently until it changes color

Meanwhile, to a small mixing dish, add hummus, chili powder, cumin, nutritional yeast, salt, and cayenne. Mix to combine. Then insert water until a pourable sauce is formed. Now add parsley and blend. Add the spice mixture in the tofu and continue to cook on medium heat until its slightly browned

Roll out a big tortilla. Add substantial portions of the roasted vegetables, scrambled tofu, avocado, cilantro, and a little salsa. Roll up and put seam side down. Continue until all toppings are being used.

Spicy Breakfast Fajitas with Eggs and Guacamole

Ingredients

- 6 ounces of avocado
- 1 tablespoon of lime juice
- Kosher salt for taste

Vegetables

- 1 tablespoon of extra-virgin olive oil
- 2 bell peppers (Red, Orange & Yellow), cut into ½-inch-wide strips
- Half white onion, medium sliced into ½-inch-wide wedges
- 1 teaspoon of ground cumin
- Half teaspoon of chili powder
- 1 Pinch red pepper flakes
- 2 garlic cloves, minced
- 2 teaspoons of fresh lime juice
- Fajitas and Garnishes

- 6 corn tortillas
- 6 eggs large
- 1 ounce of crumbled feta
- A handful of fresh cilantro, sliced
- black pepper (Freshly ground)
- Hot sauce

Preparation:

From using a spoon, scoop the flesh of the avocados into a small dish.

Insert the lime juice and 1/4 teaspoon of salt and beat with a pastry cutter, potato beater, or fork until the mixture is blended

In a large pot, heat the olive oil on medium heat.

Once the oil is sparkling, add the bell peppers and onion, cumin, chili powder, red pepper flakes, and a few pinches of salt. Toss to mix, shield the pan, and sauté, frequently stirring, until the vegetables are easily sliced by a fork, 5 to 8 minutes.

Uncover and continue cooking, Stir in between, until the vegetables are slightly well-cooked on the edges, about 3 to 5 minutes more.

Add garlic, mix well, and sauté for another minute.

Take the pan from the heat and sprinkle the lime juice. Toss, flavor to taste with additional salt, and cover to keep warm.

In the meantime, prepare the fajitas:

In a small pot on medium heat, heat each tortilla on both sides until heated well. Stack the heated tortillas on a plate as they are done and cover them with a kitchen cloth to keep warm.

Sponge the pot, spray with oil on medium-low heat.

Cautiously crack an egg and add it into the pot without breaking the yolk. Saute covered till the whites set, about 2 minutes, or longer to taste.

Move the eggs to a plate and repeat with the remaining eggs.

Spread the guacamole on each tortilla, top each with an egg, followed by some vegetables. Drizzle with cheese, cilantro, and freshly ground pepper.

Banana and Chocolate Chip Baked Oatmeal Cups

Ingredients

- 3 cups rolled oats ½ teaspoon ground cinnamon
- Half teaspoon of ground nutmeg
- 1 teaspoon of baking powder
- ¼ teaspoon of salt
- 2 eggs large
- ¼ cup of pure maple syrup
- 1 cup of mashed banana (2 bananas)
- 2 teaspoons of pure vanilla extract
- 1 cup of 1% of milk
- ¼ cup of melted coconut oil
- 1 cup of mini chocolate chips
- Cooking spray.

Preparation

Preheat the cooking oven to a temperature of 350.

Take a medium bowl, add the rolled oats, cinnamon, nutmeg, baking powder, and salt and combine.

Break the 2 eggs into another medium bowl. Mix with the mashed banana, maple syrup, and vanilla extract until the ingredients are mixed and smooth.

Slowly beat in the milk and coconut oil.

Pour the misty materials into the dry elements. Stir until all the oats are well-moistened

Slowly mix in the chocolate chips.

Sprinkle a muffin pan with cooking spray then distribute the oatmeal mixture among the 12 muffins tins. Press the mixture down with a spoon, so all the oats are covered in fluid.

Cook for about 30 minutes or till the tops are lightly brown.

"Chocolate Chia Overnight Oats"

Ingredients

- 1 cup of rolled oats
- 3 tablespoons of cocoa powder
- 1 tablespoon of chia seeds
- A pinch of salt
- 1/4 cup of Greek yogurt
- 1 cup of almond milk, unsweetened
- 2 tablespoons of maple syrup
- 1 teaspoon of vanilla extract

Preparation

First, combine dry ingredients in a dish. Now add all the wet ingredients and combine them again.

Place it in a refrigerator, make sure it is covered, for at least 2 hours or overnight. Serve cold.

Top with yogurt and fresh strawberries and enjoy the breakfast

OATMEAL BLUEBERRY YOGURT PANCAKES

Ingredients

- Half cup of rolled oats (gluten-free)
- Half teaspoon of baking powder
- 1 container of "5.3 oz." siggi's blueberry or vanilla bean yogurt
- Half banana (medium ripe)
- 1 egg
- Half teaspoon of vanilla
- 1/3 cup of fresh or frozen blueberries, Also one more to serve.

Preparation

Put all the ingredients except fresh blueberries into a mixer; mix until everything becomes smooth. Also, add a teaspoon or two of almond milk to make the batter thinner.

Place batter aside and allow it to thicken up for about a few minutes. If it is too thin, add one tablespoon or two of oats and mix again

Slightly coat a medium-sized nonstick pan or cook with butter or cooking spray and heat on a medium to low heat. Pour batter by 1/4 cup in a pan. Now add a few blueberries on the top. Prepare until bubbles started to show up. Now start flipping the cakes and cook until it changes color. Clean the pan and repeat the same procedure by sprinkling a cooking spray and leftover batter. You can easily make 4-5 pancakes.

Protein-Packed Breakfast Acron Squash

Ingredients

- Medium acorn squash (01)
- 2 teaspoons of coconut oil
- Half teaspoon of cinnamon
- 2 teaspoons of brown sugar
- 1 cup of nonfat plain Greek yogurt
- 2 teaspoons of honey
- 2 tablespoons sliced pecans

Preparation

Preheat oven to a temperature of 400 degrees F. Stripe a baking sheet with a foil.

Now chop acorn squash, half in lengthwise, and scrape the seeds out.

Take a small bowl and combine coconut oil and cinnamon. With the help of your fingers, scrub each half of the surface of the acorn squash with coconut oil and cinnamon mixture.

Put 1 teaspoon of brown sugar in between each half and scrub into the squash. Bake for around 45-60 minutes or until it becomes fork-tender.

Once squash is done, let it cool for 5-10 minutes, then serve on plates or put in the refrigerator if you are thinking of enjoying this later.

Once it's ready to serve, make sure that it is warm and scoop half cup yogurt into each squash half. Sprinkle each with a teaspoon of honey and pecans. Serve & Enjoy!

"Protein-Packed Rainbow Breakfast"

Ingredients

- Half cup cottage cheese (low fat)
- 1/4 cup of granola of your choice
- Half banana
- Half cup of strawberry slices
- Half kiwi, sliced
- 1/4 cup of blueberries
- 1 tablespoon of chia seeds
- Drizzle of cinnamon

Preparation

Add cottage cheese to a container or place in a jar. Now add granola, fruit & chia seeds. Serve & Enjoy

"Peanut Butter Energy Bites"

Ingredients

- 2/3 cup of creamy peanut butter
- Half cup of semi-sweet chocolate chips
- 1 cup oats (old fashioned)
- Half cup ground of flax seeds
- 2 tablespoons of honey

Preparation

Add all 5 ingredients in a medium-sized bowl. Mix to combine them. Put it in the refrigerator for about 15-30 minutes, so they become easier to roll.

Roll them into 12 bites and stock in the fridge for up to a week.

"Banana Pan-Cakes"

Ingredients

- 2 medium-sized ripe banana
- 2 medium-sized eggs
- Butter or oil for the saucepan

Optional ingredients:

- 2 to 3 tablespoons of almond meal
- 1 tablespoon of cocoa powder or protein powder
- 1/4 teaspoon of baking powder for fluffy pancakes
- 1/4 teaspoon of vanilla
- 1/4 cup of chocolate chips or fresh berries
- dash of cinnamon

Preparation:

Skin the banana and break it up into several big pieces in a bowl. Smoothly mash the bananas into smaller pieces using a fork. Add the eggs to the mashed bananas and stir until you have a custard-like mixture. The batter will be a bit thin and should have a few pieces of bananas. (optional: add 1/4 teaspoon of baking powder, 1/4 teaspoon of vanilla, a dash of cinnamon, 1 tablespoon of coco-powder)

Heat a grill on medium heat and Liquefy in about 1/4 teaspoon of butter in the saucepan. Put the batter on a hot grill: Drop roughly around 2 tablespoons of batter onto the hot grill. This would be a perfect time to add the nuts, chocolate chips or berries if wished.

Saute for around 1 minute or until the bottom changes color and becomes golden when you lift an edge.

Slightly flip the pancakes and cook for about a minute on the other side. Shift the cooked pancakes to a serving plate and keep on cooking the rest of the batter.

Serve these pancakes warm; they are delicious when eaten fresh off the grill and still warm. Serve with honey, maple syrup, or any extra toppings.

"Protein Pancakes"

Ingredients:

- Eggs (02)
- 2 scoops of "Whey Protein powder."
- 1 teaspoon of Baking powder
- 6 Tablespoons of Water or Almond milk
- Cooking spray, butter, or coconut oil for lubricating the pan

Preparation

Place a non-stick pan on the stove on medium heat. Drizzle with cooking spray or use butter or coconut oil and let it melt.

Combine the eggs, protein powder, and baking powder in a large-sized bowl. Add the water or almond milk in a little quantity at a time until the batter has pancake batter consistency. You might not need all of the water.

Using a 1/3 cup portion, pour out the batter into the pan.

Serve with chocolate chips, butter, and sugar-free syrup.

"Low-Calorie Ice cream."

Ingredients

- 1 A cup of unsweetened Almond or dairy-free milk
- 3 tablespoon of Gelatin
- 6 cups of ice
- 1 tablespoon of Coconut oil
- 1 teaspoon of Vanilla
- Seasoned Stevia
- Dash of Salt

Preparation:

Heat the milk in a skillet until it reaches a light boil

Transfer the gelatin on warm milk in a thin layer and stir until it is completely softened.

Place in a food mixer and blend on high. Add remaining ingredients except for ice.

After it gets slightly frothy (about 30 seconds in), slowly start adding one cube at a time.

If the mix stalls at any time, pulse the food mixture.

Sometimes the mix will cluster and becomes jelly. If that's the case, just add more water and ice.

You can continue to mix it until you find the right mixture. More gelatin will make it denser. More oil will make it smoother. More almond milk makes it more of a Frostie.

Be patient with mixing. It can take a while, depending on the quality of your mixer.

"Egg Muffins"

Ingredients

- 1/4 cup of sun-dried tomatoes, cubed
- Half cup of spinach
- 6 eggs
- 3 egg whites
- Dash of salt
- coconut oil (Spray)
- any other veggies you like

Preparation:

Drizzle mini muffin tins with coconut oil spray.

Mix eggs and egg whites in a bowl and beat to combine. Cut spinach and sun-dried tomatoes and add to the mixture.

Now add the egg mixture into muffin tins, ensuring to scoop the sun-dried tomatoes and spinach into each muffin tin as well.

Bake for around 20-25 minutes.

Store in a sealed container after the eggs have cooled. It can be used for up to 04 days!

"Protein Brownie in a Mug"

Ingredients

- 1/4 cup of almond milk
- 1/4 teaspoon of vanilla extract
- 1 scoop of chocolate protein powder
- One and a half tablespoon of unsweetened cocoa powder
- Half tablespoon of coconut flour
- Half teaspoon of baking powder
- 5 to 10 drops of liquid stevia (depending on your taste) or any other available sweetener

Preparation

Whisk together all of the ingredients. Discharge into a mug. Heat in the microwave for about 25-35 seconds, or until the middle is cake-like and the top and edges are slightly running.

"Cinnamon Roll French Toast Casserole"

Ingredients

French Toast

- 1 loaf "12 slices" sourdough bread, divided into 1-inch cubes (~6 cups)
- 8 large-sized eggs
- 1 cup of milk, any type
- 1 teaspoon of vanilla extract
- 2 tablespoons of maple syrup
- Half cup of walnuts, crushed

Almond Butter Cinnamon Drizzle

- 2/3 cup of almond butter, drippy
- 2 tablespoons of maple syrup
- 3 teaspoons of ground cinnamon
- 1 tablespoon of melted coconut oil

Optional Topping

- 4 tablespoons of butter, chilled

- 1/4 cup of brown sugar

Preparation:

Drizzle a 7 – 8-inch glass bowl with coconut oil cooking spray. In this bowl, you will use to cook your French toast in. Place it aside.

Next, take a small bowl whisk together all the ingredients for the almond butter cinnamon sprinkle. The consistency should be soft, and if it's not, add more coconut oil.

Take a medium-sized bowl, add eggs, milk, vanilla, and maple syrup.

Place half of the bread cubes and half of the walnuts in the glass container. Sprinkle on half of the almond butter cinnamon drizzle over bread combination. Add the remaining bread cubes and drizzle on the remaining walnuts and cinnamon sprinkle over the bread.

Add egg mixture over the entire thing and mix bread cubes with the egg mixture with the help of a spatula. Then, drizzle on the optional topping.

Position metal Instant Pot trivet on the bottom of Instant Pot and pour in 1 cup of water. Then, place a French toast container on top of the trivet.

Lock Instant Pot and move pressure valve to closure. Press manual and move to high pressure and cook for about 25 minutes.

Now release and remove Instant Pot cover. Allow it to cool and then serve with fruit and maple syrup.

"Matcha Glazed Donuts"

Ingredients:

- Half cup of vanilla Tone It Up Protein
- Half cup of gluten-free oat flour
- 1 teaspoon of baking powder
- Half teaspoon of ground cinnamon
- Dash of salt
- 1/4 cup of unsweetened almond milk
- 1/4 cup of maple syrup
- 1 medium-sized egg
- 1 teaspoon of vanilla extract
- 1 tablespoon of coconut oil, melted
- Coconut oil spray

Glaze:

- 1 cup of unsweetened almond or coconut yogurt
- 1 teaspoon of matcha

Preparation:

Preheat oven to a temperature of 350 degrees.

Mix all dry ingredients in a bowl and beat to combine

Take a separate bowl, mix all wet ingredients.

Add the wet ingredients in the dry ones and stir to mix them

Sprinkle a donut pan with coconut oil spray and add batter. Bake for about 15-20 minutes or until a toothpick comes out clean.

For the glaze, beat ingredients together in a small-sized bowl. Mix donuts in glaze.

Chapter 03: Best Quick & Easy Recipes to Lose Weight (Lunch)

Indian Shrimp Curry

Ingredients:

- 1 tablespoon of canola oil, separate
- 1 pound of shrimp, skinned and deveined
- Half yellow onion, nicely chopped
- 1 teaspoon of ground ginger
- 1 teaspoon of ground cumin
- 1 teaspoon of ground coriander
- One and a half teaspoon of ground turmeric
- 1 teaspoon of curry powder
- 1 teaspoon of paprika
- Half teaspoon of chili powder
- Garlic cloves (02), crushed
- 15 ounce can of tomato sauce
- 3/4 cup of lite canned coconut milk

- Half teaspoon of Kosher salt
- cilantro and chili peppers for garnishing

Preparation:

Add 2 teaspoons of the canola oil over high heat in a large pan.

Now add the shrimp and cook for about a minute on each side then take the shrimp out of the pan.

Insert the remaining teaspoon of the canola oil to the pan with the onions.

Prepare the onions for about 5 minutes over medium heat, stirring irregularly.

Add the cumin, coriander, ginger, turmeric, paprika, chili powder, curry powder, salt, and garlic.

Mix them well, let it cook for 30 seconds and add the tomato sauce and combine.

Add in the coconut milk and shrimp to the skillet and mix well.

Decorate with cilantro and chili peppers if wished.

ROAST BEEF AND HORSE RADISH

Ingredients:

- 2 tablespoons "2% plain" Greek yogurt
- 1 tablespoon of horseradish sauce
- Bibb lettuce (2 leaves)
- 4 pieces lean deli-style roast beef
- 4 slices of tomato
- 1 cup of fresh raspberries

Preparation:

Mix yogurt and horseradish, and spread it on lettuce. On the top, add roast beef and tomato and roll into a wrap. Your lunch is ready to be served with raspberries.

Tuna Avocado Sandwich

Ingredients:

- 1/3 avocado, smashed
- Half tablespoon of lemon juice
- 4 oz. white albacore tuna, drained
- 1 thick slice of tomato
- 1 piece of butter lettuce
- 1 slice of red onion
- 1 slice of whole-grain bread

Preparation:

Mix avocado with lemon juice and wrap in tuna. Pile tomato, lettuce, onion, and avocado and tuna mixture on a piece of bread for an open-face sandwich.

Pepper and Onion Wraps

Ingredients

- 1 tablespoon of extra-virgin olive oil
- 2 medium sliced bell peppers (green)
- 1 medium sweet onion thinly sliced
- Half eggplant, small & sliced
- Half teaspoon of kosher or sea salt
- 2 tablespoons of grated parmesan cheese
- 2 pieces of whole-grain tortillas
- 2 dashes of hot sauce

Preparation

In a medium-sized saucepan, heat olive oil on a medium to low heat and insert onions, peppers, and eggplant. Cook for about 10 minutes or until it changes color.

Slightly heat tortillas in a pan on a medium to high heat for about 30 seconds each side.

Steadily add veggies on a warm tortilla; add a pinch of salt, parmesan, and a dash of hot sauce.

Wrap it up and enjoy the meal!

Salmon & Avocado Salad with Lemon Dressing

Ingredients

For "Salmon & Avocado Salad"

- 1 "6 to 8 ounce" can of wild salmon
- 1 avocado, skinned and cubed
- 2 cups of salad greens (loosely packed)
- Half cup of reduced-fat Monterey jack (in shreds)
- 3/4 cup of tomato (chopped)
- 1 tablespoon of freshly squeezed lemon juice (half lemon)

"Lemon Dressing"

- 1 tablespoon of freshly squeezed lemon juice (half lemon)
- 1 tablespoon of extra-virgin olive oil
- 1 teaspoon of honey
- 1/8 teaspoon of kosher or sea salt

- 1/8 teaspoon of black pepper
- Half teaspoon of Dijon mustard
- 2 jars for storage

Preparation

Beat together all the ingredients for the salad dressing except olive oil. Gently sprinkle olive oil, beating all the while. The dressing can be done separately or positioned as the first ingredient in the bottom of the jars.

Mix avocado in lemon juice. It will add some vitality to the avocado and keep it from toasting.

Now add an even amount of chopped tomatoes in each jar, then add cheese, then add avocado, then add salmon, and finally lettuce. Tightly screw the lid on jars and refrigerate until it is ready to eat.

Lemon Pepper Salmon Caesar Salad

Ingredients

For dressing:

- Half cup of plain Greek yogurt
- 2 tablespoons of grated Parmesan cheese
- 2 tablespoons of olive oil
- Lemon juice (from 1 lemon)
- 1 teaspoon of Dijon mustard
- Garlic Clove 01
- Anchovy filets 01 (optional)

For Salad:

- 2 heads of Romaine lettuce, chopped
- 2 ounces of Parmesan cheese, peeled with a vegetable peeler
- Salmon:
- 2 teaspoons of freshly ground black pepper

- 3/4 teaspoon of sea salt
- 2 teaspoons of lemon zest
- 4-6 ounces of salmon filets
- 2 tablespoons of olive oil

Preparation

For the dressing: Put all the ingredients in mixer and beat until it becomes smooth.

For the salad: Add Romaine lettuce and peeled cheese in a large-sized bowl. Mix with dressing and make sure it is well coated.

For salmon:

Mix black pepper, salt, and lemon zest in a small-sized bowl until they are well-combined. Coat salmon fillets with flavors. Put a heavy cast iron or stainless steel pan on the stove. Turn to medium to high heat. Heat the pan for about 3-4 minutes, or until very hot, now add oil. When the oil starts boiling, add fish to skillet 1-2 fillets at one time.

Cook until the fish lifts easily with a spatula (if it doesn't, leave it there until it lifts with no effort. Start flipping, and continue cooking until fish changes color on both sides and flakes with the help of a fork. Now cook the remaining fillets.

Avocado & Grape Salad with Walnuts

Ingredients

- 1 avocado, peeled, sliced and pitted
- 2 tablespoons of freshly-squeezed lemon juice (from one lemon),
- One and a half cup of halved-grapes
- 1/3 cup of coarsely sliced walnuts
- Half cup of celery (thinly sliced)
- 1 package of baby arugula or kale
- 1 green apple, cored, sliced, and divided
- 1/4 teaspoon kosher or sea salt
- 1/4 teaspoon of black pepper

Preparation

Mix avocado slices with one tablespoon of lemon juice. Mix apple slices separately with a remaining tablespoon of lemon juice. Now add grapes, walnuts, celery, apple, baby kale or arugula, and salt and pepper altogether. Cautiously add avocado and toss again.

Enjoy the lunch with your favorite clean eating salad dressing or vinaigrette served mixed in a salad or on the side.

SKINNY BURRITO IN A JAR

Ingredients

- 1 cup of salsa (without Sugar)
- 1 "15 ounces" can of beans (black), drained
- 1 cup of reduced-fat cheddar cheese, in shreds
- Half cup Greek Yogurt, non-fat

Preparation

Equally, divide every ingredient into 4 (Half pint size) canning jars. Add ingredients as per the order: 1/4 cup of salsa, 1/4 heaping cup of black beans, 1/4 cup of cheese, and 2 tablespoons of yogurt or sour cream.

Refrigerate the jar for up to two days. After two days, have it straight from the jar or add to a whole wheat wrap.

TIP: Try to add 1/4 cup of cooked quinoa or brown rice in each jar.

PROTEIN COBB SALAD WITH QUINOA

Ingredients

- 6 cups baby lettuce (loosely packed) any variety
- 2 eggs, full boiled, halved and peeled
- One and a half cup of halved cherry or grape tomatoes
- 1 avocado, diced, peeled, and pitted
- 1 cup of uncooked quinoa of any brand
- 1/4 cup of olive oil
- Lemon Juice (From 1 lemon)
- 1 teaspoon of Dijon mustard
- 1/4 teaspoon of kosher or sea salt
- 1/4 teaspoon of black pepper

Preparation

Start cooking quinoa by adding it to a bowl with 1-1/4 cups of water and a drizzle of salt. Cook on high heat, and uncovered, until it boils. Mix once and cover again. Now reduce the heat to the lowest level. Allow it to cook for about

20 to 25 minutes or until the water is completely absorbed. Uncover and fluff with a fork.

To thoroughly boil the eggs, place them in a small pot, and cover with an inch of cold water. Bring it to a boil over medium heat. Cover and remove from the temperature. Allow it to cool for 10 minutes. Peel and cut them in halves.

Mix the juice of lemon and Dijon mustard. Add olive oil in a slow and balanced stream, start beating all this while until combined. Beat in salt and pepper.

Mix lettuce and cherry tomatoes.

Top it in the order: cooked quinoa first, then eggs, and avocado in the last

Garnish it on the sides and enjoy the meal.

Sprouts, Veggies, and Cheese Wrap

Ingredients

- 1/4 cup of grated carrots
- Half cup of shredded romaine lettuce
- Half cucumber, in round parts, then in halves
- Half cup of bean sprouts
- Half cup of cubed tomatoes
- 1/8 cup of chopped red onions (it's optional)
- 1/4 cup of part-skim mozzarella (shredded), low-fat Monterrey, or cheddar cheese (low fat)
- 1/4 cup of clean eating dressing or spread of choice, like hummus or guacamole homemade or store, bought
- 1 complete wheat or spinach wrap (large)

Preparation

Place the wraps. Equally, distribute the dressing or spread, leave about 2-inches on one end to fold. Now add a uniform layer of cheese and all of the fillings to each wrap. Fold it over and tuck in on the bottom.

Creamy Sweet Potato and Pear Soup

Ingredients

- Half cup of onions (chopped)

- Garlic clove 01, crushed

- 1 tablespoon of fresh thyme leaves

- 5 cups of vegetable or chicken stock

- 2 pears of any variety, chopped, cored, and peeled

- 3/4 cup of sliced celery

- 2 large carrots, chopped and skinned

- 2 sweet potatoes, chopped and skinned

- 1 cup of low fat (2%) plain Greek yogurt, (optional)

- 1 tablespoon of olive oil

- 1 teaspoon of turmeric

- 1/16 (a pinch) of teaspoon nutmeg

- 2 tablespoons of coconut palm sugar or honey

- 1 tablespoon of freshly squeezed lemon juice (From half lemon)

- Half teaspoon of salt

Preparation

Pour olive oil to the bottom of a heavy-bottomed soup container on medium heat. Add onions, celery, carrots, and start cooking until onions are soft and radiant, but other vegetables don't need to be soft.

Add the turmeric powder and garlic and start cooking for an extra 30 seconds, stirring. Add the broth, sweet potatoes, pears, and salt and mix well. Also, add in the sweetener. Keep on cooking on a medium to low heat; allow it to boil for around 30 to 40 minutes until the vegetables become soft. Remove from the heat.

Crush until it becomes smooth in a blender, fill only halfway every time, start the blender on low and hold the top with a kitchen towel. Add extra broth or lemon juice if a solvent consistency is required. Add the nutmeg, and start stirring. Now add lemon juice and stir. Beat in the Greek yogurt, if you are using it until mixed well.

Decorate it with thyme sprigs or sliced parsley to serve, if wished. Enjoy the meal!

Lentil & Kale Soup

Ingredients

- 1 medium onion, chopped (coarsely)
- 1 tablespoon of extra-virgin olive oil
- 1 medium-sized carrot, coarsely chopped & peeled
- 1 stalk of celery, chopped (coarsely)
- 1 cup of kale (chopped)
- Half cup of lentils
- 3 cups of vegetable broth
- 2 bay leaves, torn in half
- 2 cups of canned lite coconut milk
- Half teaspoon of salt
- Half teaspoon of pepper
- 1 cup of water "to water it down."

Preparation

On medium to low heat, in a skillet with extra-virgin olive oil, cook the onions for about 2 minutes and add the carrots and celery. Cook them for about 5 minutes.

Add the kale and start cooking for another 10 minutes.

Add the lentils then start tossing them in the skillet for about 2 min.

Add the bay leaves and vegetable broth. Allow it to simmer on low heat for about 20 minutes.

Add the coconut milk and start cooking for another 10 minutes.

Flavor with salt and pepper, then take away the bay leaves and remove them.

By using the immersion blender, blend the soup until it becomes smooth and creamy.

Start cooking for another 5 minutes. Change the consistency of the soup with the water.

Scoop them to individual mugs then sprinkle with extra virgin olive oil.

Avocado Chicken Wrap

Ingredients

- 2 pieces of chicken breast, on the bone
- 2 teaspoons of extra-virgin olive oil
- Half teaspoon of kosher or sea salt
- Half teaspoon of black pepper
- Half teaspoon of chili powder
- 1 avocado ripped, pitted, peeled and chopped
- 1 tablespoon of freshly-squeezed lime juice
- 1 cup of quartered cherry tomatoes
- 4 scallions (sliced)
- 2 cups of bibb lettuce (chopped), optional romaine heart
- 1 "15-ounce" can of refried beans
- Half cup of salsa, without sugar
- 8 "8-inch", whole grain tortillas

Preparation

Preheat oven to a temperature of 350 degrees.

Wash chicken breasts and pat dry with a paper towel. Coat chicken with olive oil and drizzle with 1/4 teaspoon of salt, 1/4 teaspoon of pepper, and chili powder. Place in an oven-safe skillet, cover, and bake for 1 hour, or until juices trip clear when pierced with a fork.

Take the chicken from the oven and allow it to cool until it is easy to handle. Get rid of skin and discard.

Take the chicken from the bone and shred into small strips, by using a fork or just hands.

As the chicken is cooling, mash it with a fork, sliced avocado, remaining salt and pepper, and a lime juice. Add refried beans into a skillet, place on a medium to low heat, and start cooking until its hot.

Heat tortillas on a dry pan on medium heat, for about 01 minutes each side, or just until warmed thoroughly. Spread over the warm tortillas, small amounts of refried beans, salsa, lettuce, shredded pieces of chicken, tomatoes, and scallions. Top each side with mashed avocado mixture. Fold the end under and roll each wrap to serve. Enjoy the meal!

Possible toppings: Greek yogurt or sour cream, minced cheddar cheese.

Japanese Tuna Salad

Ingredients

- 2 "6-ounce" cans of tuna, drained and peeled
- Half cup of plain Greek yogurt
- Lemon Juice (from 1 lemon)
- 1 small onion, chopped
- jalapeño pepper (01), seeded and chopped
- 1 avocado, pitted, cubed, and peeled
- 1/4 cup of freshly chopped cilantro
- Half teaspoon of sea salt
- 1/4 teaspoon of fresh ground pepper (black)
- 4 cups of baby spinach leaves

Preparation

Mix all the ingredients except for the spinach in a large-sized bowl. Combine well and chill until it is ready to serve. Then serve the tuna salad over the spinach leaves.

Asian Chicken & Veggie Lettuce Wraps

Ingredients

- 1 pound of skinless, boneless pieces of chicken breasts, sliced into strips
- 2 tablespoons of canola oil
- Half bell pepper (red), sliced into strips
- 1-inch of knob ginger root, minced and peeled
- Garlic Cloves 02, crushed
- 1 medium-sized carrot, sliced and peeled into thin strips

- For the dressing purpose
- 2 tablespoons of sesame oil
- 1/3 cup of rice wine vinegar
- 2 tablespoons of lite soy sauce, (optional Tamari or coconut aminos)
- 1 tablespoon sesame seeds, brown

- 1/16 teaspoon of cayenne pepper (it's optional)

For serving purpose

- large butter lettuce leaves (06), washed and dried
- 2 green onions, minced

Preparation

Crisp sesame seeds in a dry skillet on a low to medium heat for around 1 to 2 minutes, constantly stir or just until it changes color. Then set aside.

For the Dressing:

In a medium-sized bowl, beat together the dressing ingredients.

Add 1 tablespoon of canola oil to a large skillet on medium heat. Once the oil is hot "shimmering but not smoking," add chicken strips into it. Start cooking until the chicken turns golden from all sides and cooked well. Take out chicken strips and set aside. Add to the pan the remaining oil, carrots, red pepper strips, and ginger. Start cooking until veggies are only lightly tender and still crispy. In the last 30 seconds, add the crushed garlic and cook just until you smell the fragrance. Add chicken again to the pan with the veggies and add dressing, toss to mix.

To assemble:

Bring together wraps by laying down lettuce leaf, and add the chicken and veggies. Top each wrap with chopped green onions.

Chapter 04: Deliciously Healthy Dinner Recipes for Weight Loss

Rosemary Citrus One Pan Baked Salmon

Ingredients:

- 1/3 cup of olive oil
- Ground pepper (a pinch)
- 2 tablespoon of fresh orange juice
- 2 tablespoon of fresh rosemary. Also, 1-2 extra sprigs to garnish
- 1 tablespoon of Lemon juice
- Half teaspoon of garlic crushed
- 1/4 teaspoon of grated dried orange peel (sliced)
- Kosher salt or fine sea salt to add flavor
- 1 bunch of thin asparagus (trimmed) (Or any other vegetable of your choice)
- Olive oil or melted butter to sprinkle
- "10–12" ounces of sockeye salmon (whole fillet or about 3 fillets)

- 5-6 oranges thinly sliced

- Optional ingredient:

- 1/4 teaspoon of lemon pepper

- Additional Salt/pepper to add flavor – after baking

Preparation:

Preheating oven up to a temperature of 400 degrees F.

Mix orange juice, lemon, 2 tablespoons of rosemary, 1/4 to 1/3 cup of olive oil, a pinch of salt, pepper, 1/4 teaspoon of orange peel, and garlic. Set them aside.

Next, make a layer on a dish

First of all, add trimmed asparagus or any other vegetable and sprinkle with olive oil or butter. Add one pinch (1/4 teaspoon or so) of lemon pepper flavor.

Place salmon (skin side down) between the asparagus spears.

Sprinkle the orange rosemary marinade on top of salmon.

Now add thin slices of orange on top of salmon and asparagus.

Put 2 to 2 fresh sprigs of rosemary equally on top of the salmon and around the pot.

Drizzle a bit more orange peel, pepper, and kosher salt on top of the salmon veggie bake.

Bake it at 400F for about 12-15 minutes or until salmon is no longer opaque in the middle.

Nutrition per serving: 345 calories in total, 22 g of fat (3 g sat), 25 g of protein, 10 g of carb, 5 g of sugars, 3 g of fiber

Mushroom and Black Bean Smothered Burritos

Ingredients:

- 100 g "~ 1/3 cup" of white rice
- 1 tablespoon of oil
- 1 medium-sized onion, diced or sliced
- 8 medium mushrooms, diced or sliced
- 2 garlic cloves, crushed
- 2 teaspoons of smoked paprika
- 1 teaspoon of ground cumin
- 1 tablespoon of tomato puree or paste
- 145 g "~ 2/3 cup" of black beans cooked "~ 3/4 of a standard tin."
- Salt to add flavor
- Black pepper to add flavor
- 4 large-sized flour tortillas

- 150 g of cheddar cheese, grated "~ 1 1/2 cups when grated."

- 1 tablespoon of pickled jalapeños (I used green), finely minced

- 1 tablespoon of coriander (cilantro), finely minced

- 3 tablespoons of sour cream

Additional Toppings to serve (optional): chopped tomatoes, minced red onion, black olives, fresh coriander, jalapeños, diced avocado, etc.

Preparation:

Start boiling the rice in plenty of water until they are well-cooked, then drain.

Meanwhile, start heating a dash of oil in a large-sized frying pan, and add onions and mushrooms. Start cooking for about a few minutes on medium heat until lightly softened, now add the garlic, cumin, smoked paprika, and tomato puree. Cook them for a few extra minutes, stirring frequently.

Now add the black beans and the cooked rice and flavor generously. Mix them well to combine.

Take one of the large-sized flour tortillas, and add around 1/4 of the rice mixture to the center. Top it with 1/4 of the grated cheese. Crease two sides of the tortilla inside, then revolve through 90° and crease in the other two sides to fully wrap the burrito.

Repeat the same procedure with the residual tortillas, rice, and cheese, and put the burritos seam-side down on a baking dish.

Take a small bowl, combine the finely sliced jalapeños, coriander, and sour cream. Flavor with a pinch of salt and pepper, and mix them well.

Spread the sour cream sauce over the 4 burritos, and divide it around a little. Bake at a temperature of 375 degrees F for about 15-20 minutes, or until its crisped up to your liking. Now serve with the additional toppings of your choice.

Nutrition per serving: 486 calories in total, 22 g of fat (10.7 g sat), 18.7 g of protein, 53 g of carb, 665 mg of sodium, 3 g of sugars, 5.4 g of fiber

Arroz Con Pollo, Lightened Up.

Ingredients:

- 8 pieces of skinless chicken thighs
- 1 tablespoon of vinegar
- 2 teaspoons of Sazon, homemade or Badia Sazon (Tropical)
- Half teaspoon of adobo powder, Goya
- Half tablespoon of garlic powder
- 3 teaspoons of olive oil
- Half small sized onion
- 1/4 cup of cilantro
- 3 garlic cloves
- Scallions (05)
- 2 tablespoons of bell pepper
- 1 medium-sized vine tomato, chopped
- 2 & a half cups of enriched long-grain white rice
- 4 cups of water

- 1 chicken of bouillon cube
- kosher salt to add flavor, around 2 teaspoons

Preparation:

Flavor chicken with vinegar, half teaspoon of season, adobo and garlic powder and let it sit for about 10 minutes.

Start heating a large deep heavy pan on medium heat, and add 2 teaspoons of oil when it is hot.

Add chicken and cook it for about 5 minutes every side. Remove and place them aside.

Place garlic, scallions, onion, cilantro, and pepper in a small food processor. Add remaining teaspoons of olive oil to the pan and cook onion mixture on medium to low until it is soft around 3 minutes.

Add tomato, cook for an additional one minute. Add rice, mix them well, and cook for one more minute.

Add water, bouillon (Make sure it dissolves well), and the remaining season, now scratching up any browned bits from the bottom of the pan.

Taste it to check salt, should taste salty enough to suit your choice, add more if needed.

Add chicken and settle into rice, bring it to a boil. Boil it on medium to low until most of the water evaporates and liquid starts to make bubble at the top of the rice line, then reduce temperature to low heat and cover it. Make sure the lid has a fine seal, and no steam should escape. "You could place a tin foil or paper towel in between the lid and the pan if steam evaporates."

Cook for around 20 minutes without opening the lid. Turn the heat off and let it sit with the lid on for an additional 10 minutes. Enjoy!

Nutrition per serving: 410 calories in total, 8 g of fat (2 g sat), 33.5 g of protein, 47 g of carb, 655mg of sodium, 0.5 g of sugars, 1 g of fiber

Healthy Greek Chicken and Farro Salad

Ingredients:

- 1 and 1/4 cup of quick-cooking farro
- 2 tablespoons of olive oil
- Half small-sized red onion, finely sliced
- 4 tablespoon of lemon juice
- Kosher salt and pepper to add flavor
- 12 oz. of boneless, skinless chicken breasts, sliced around ½ inch thick
- 1/4 cup of fresh dill, minced
- 8 oz. of grape tomatoes, sliced
- Half of the seedless cucumber, sliced into ½-inch pieces
- 3 oz. of baby arugula (about 3 cups)
- 3 oz. of feta, crushed

Preparation:

Start cooking farro as per directions mentioned on the package, then drain, shift to a large-sized bowl, and start tossing with 1 tablespoon of oil.

Meanwhile, take a small bowl, toss onion with 2 tablespoons of lemon juice and a pinch of salt. Let them sit and toss twice.

Now heat the remaining tablespoons of oil in a large pot on medium-high. Flavor chicken with ¼ tsp of each salt and pepper and cook until it changes color, about 8 to 10 minutes.

Remove the pot from temperature and stir in the remaining 2 tablespoons of lemon juice.

Now add chicken and other juices to farro along with cucumber, dill, tomatoes, and onion (and their juices); toss them to combine. Fold it in arugula and feta.

Nutrition per serving: 380 calories in total, 10 g of fat (1.5 g sat), 26 g of protein, 198 mg of sodium, 44 g of carb, 4 g of sugar (0 g added sugar), 7 g of fiber

Instant Pot Beef and Barley Stew

Ingredients:

- 1 lb. of beef chuck, well-trimmed, sliced into 2-inch pieces
- 1 tablespoon of flour (all-purpose)
- 1 tablespoon of olive oil
- 1 large-sized onion, minced
- 4 garlic cloves, crushed
- 8 sprigs thyme, and leaves for serving
- Kosher salt and pepper to add flavor
- 1 "12-oz" bottle of beer
- Half medium butternut squash (1 pound), seeded and peeled, sliced into 2-inch pieces
- 3 medium-sized carrots (about 12 ounces), divided
- 3 cup of no-salt-added beef broth
- 1 cup of pearled barley

Preparation:

Set instant pan to cook. In a medium-sized bowl, toss beef with the flour. Now add olive oil to the instant pan and cook beef until it changes color on all sides, about 5 to 6 minutes. Shift beef to a plate.

Now add thyme sprigs, onion, garlic, and half teaspoon of each salt and pepper and cook, infrequently stirring, until tender, about 5 to 6 minutes. Stir in beer—press cancel.

Return beef to the pan along with the beef stock, squash, carrots, and barley. Place the lid to cover and cook on high pressure for about 16 minutes. Use the quick-release method to release pressure. Serve drizzled with additional thyme if wished.

Nutrition per serving: 485 calories in total, 9 g of fat (2 g sat), 35 g of protein, 490 mg of sodium, 67 g of carb, 13 g of fiber.

Coconut-Lime Marinated Shrimp and Noodles

Ingredients:

- 3 medium-sized limes
- 3/4 cup of light coconut milk
- 1 teaspoon of low-sodium soy sauce
- 2 garlic cloves
- 1 1-inch piece of a fresh ginger
- 1 red chile
- One and a half cup of fresh cilantro
- 2 scallions, finely sliced, white and green parts separated
- 1 large-sized, thick carrot
- 2 medium-sized zucchini
- 1 red pepper, finely cubed

- 1 lb of cooked, peeled, deveined shrimp

Preparation:

Finely add the zest of one lime into a large bowl, then squeeze all limes (should yield about 1/4 cup). Beat in coconut milk and soy sauce. Slightly grate in garlic, ginger, and a half red chile. Finely chopped half cup of cilantro and stir into the bowl alongside with scallion whites. Finely slice the rest of the chile and set aside.

By using a spiralizer fixed with the finest noodle blade, spiralize the carrot, and use a larger blade to spiralize zucchini. Toss noodles with a coconut milk mixture; let it sit for about 10 minutes.

After 10 minutes, fold in shrimp, red pepper, and remaining cilantro. Drizzle with remaining scallions and sliced chile.

Nutrition per serving: 225 calories in total, 5.5 g of fat (2.5 g sat), 32 g of protein, 415 mg of sodium, 14 g of carb, 7 g of sugars, 3 g of fiber

GRILLED WATERMELON + STEAK SALAD

Ingredients:

- 1 lb of sirloin (about an inch thick)
- Kosher salt and pepper to add flavor
- 3 tablespoon of fresh lemon
- 2 tablespoon of olive oil
- 2 tablespoon of honey
- Half small-sized red onion, finely sliced
- 1 lb. of cherry tomatoes, cubed
- Half of small seedless watermelon
- 1 c. of fresh mint, leaves torn
- 1 c. of fresh flat-leaf parsley leaves
- 1 small bunch of arugula, thick stems are thrown out

Preparation:

Start heating grill on a medium to high temperature. Flavor steak with a half teaspoon of each salt and pepper and grill as per your desire (around 6-8 minutes per side for medium-rare). Shift to a cutting board and let it rest for some time before slicing.

Meanwhile, in a bowl, beat together oil, honey, lemon juice, and a pinch each salt and pepper. Fold in tomatoes and onions.

Cut watermelon into a half-inch-thick triangles and cut off the rinds. Coat lightly with oil, then grill until its lightly charred, around 1-2 minutes per side. Divide into four plates.

Fold herbs into tomato blend, then gently toss with arugula. Spoon on top of the watermelon and serve it with steak.

Nutrition per serving: 361 calories in total, 18 g of fat (4.5 g sat), 28 g of protein, 346 mg of sodium, 24 g of carb, 16 g of sugar, 4.5 g of fiber

Smashed Pea and Ricotta Pappardelle

Ingredients:

- 12 oz. of pappardelle
- One and a half c. of frozen peas, defrosted
- 1 teaspoon of lemon zest
- Half c. of part-skim ricotta cheese
- Half teaspoon of kosher salt
- Half teaspoon of pepper
- 1/4 c. of chives, minced

Preparation:

Start cooking pasta as per the directions mentioned on the package. Reserve half cup of the cooking water; drain pasta and return to skillet.

Meanwhile, pasta is cooking, pulse one cup of defrosted peas in a food processor until roughly minced. Add ricotta and zest and pulse a few times to mix, then flavor with salt and pepper.

Toss pasta with ricotta blend and remaining half cup of peas, add reserved pasta water if the pasta seems dry. Drizzle with minced chives and serve.

Nutrition per serving: 430 calories in total, 6.5 g of fat (2.5 g sat), 19 g of protein, 100 mg of sodium, 70 g of carbs, 5 g of fiber

Grilled Chicken with Smoky Corn Salad

Ingredients:

- 4 "6-oz" of boneless, skinless chicken breast halves
- Salt and Pepper to add flavor
- 2 limes, sliced
- 4 ears corn (shucked)
- 1/4 c. of cilantro, minced
- 2 tablespoons of sliced green olives
- 1 oz. of Manchego cheese, thinly grated
- One and a half teaspoon of olive oil
- 1 teaspoon of smoked paprika

Preparation:

Flavor boneless, skinless chicken-breast halves with salt and pepper and grill on medium to a high temperature to cook well, about 5 to 6 minutes on both sides.

Meanwhile, grill limes, cut it down, and corn until well-cooked, about 6 to 8 minutes.

Cut corn from the cob and toss in a bowl with the juice of 2 lime halves, then minced cilantro, sliced green olives, grated Manchego cheese, and pinch each salt and pepper.

Serve chicken with corn and remaining lime slices and sprinkle with a mixture of olive oil and smoked paprika.

Nutrition per serving: 355 calories in total, 13 g of fat (3.5 g saturated), 21 g of protein, 315 mg of sodium, 21 g of carb, 2 g of fiber

White Beans and Tuna Salad with Basil Vinaigrette

Ingredients:

- Kosher salt and pepper to add flavor
- 12 oz. of green beans, halved and trimmed
- 1 small-sized shallot, cubed
- 1 cup of lightly packed basil leaves
- 3 tablespoon of olive oil
- 1 tablespoon of red wine vinegar
- 4 cup of torn lettuce
- 1 "15-oz" can of small white beans, cleaned
- 2 "5-oz" cans of solid white tuna in water, drained
- 4 soft-boiled eggs, divided

Preparation:

Take a large pot of water and allow it to boil. Add 1 tablespoon of salt, then green beans, and start cooking until just tender, about 3 to 4 minutes. Drain and rinse under cold water and allow it to cool.

Meanwhile, in a mixer, mix shallot, basil, oil, vinegar, and half teaspoon of each salt and pepper until it is smooth.

Shift half of dressing to a large-sized bowl and toss with green beans. Fold in white beans, lettuce, and tuna and serve with remaining dressing and eggs.

Nutrition per serving: 340 calories in total, 16.5 g of fat (3 g saturated), 31 g of protein, 770 mg of sodium, 24 g of carb, 8 g of fiber

Rhubarb and Citrus Salad (Black Pepper Vinaigrette)

Ingredients:

- 2 tablespoons of honey
- 2 tablespoons of white wine vinegar
- 3 stalks rhubarb, cropped, and cut into 1-in. pieces
- 1/4 cup of olive oil
- Kosher salt and pepper to add flavor
- 2 oranges
- 3 oz. of baby spinach (about 4 c.)
- 2 bunches of watercress, thick stems detached
- 1/4 cup of toasted pistachios, crushed
- 1 oz. of Ricotta Salata (shaved)

Preparation:

Take a small bowl, beat together honey and vinegar. Add rhubarb and start tossing to coat. Let stand about 5 minutes and up to a maximum of 10 minutes, now add olive oil, half teaspoons of salt, and 2 teaspoons of coarsely ground pepper.

In the meanwhile, cut away peel and white pith from oranges, then finely slice.

In a large-sized bowl, toss spinach and watercress; fold in orange pieces and divide them among plates. Spoon rhubarb and dressing on each salad and top with pistachios and Ricotta Salata.

Nutrition per serving: 280 calories in total, 19.5 g of fat (3.5 g saturated), 5 g of protein, 380 mg of sodium, 25 g of carbohydrate, 4 g of fiber

POT STICKER STIR-FRY

Ingredients:

- 1 pack of vegetable potstickers or

- 2 tablespoons of hoisin sauce
- 2 tablespoons of fresh lime juice
- 1 tablespoon of water
- 1 tablespoon of vegetable oil
- 1 red pepper, finely cubed
- 1 yellow pepper, finely cubed
- 1 tablespoon of finely crushed fresh ginger
- 1 small-sized red onion, finely sliced
- 8 oz. of snow peas, sliced diagonally

Preparation:

Pan-fry vegetable potstickers in a large pot as the directions mentioned on the package; shift to plate. Beat together fresh lime juice, hoisin sauce, and water.

Now add vegetable oil to the pot and start heating on medium temperature. Add red pepper, yellow pepper, and thinly crushed fresh ginger and cook, frequently tossing about 5 minutes. Add small-sized red onion and cook, toss, about 1 minute.

Add snow peas and cook, shielded, frequently tossing, until vegetables are just tender, around 4 minutes. Toss vegetables with sauce and serve with potstickers.

Nutrition per serving: 240 calories in total, 6.5 g of fat (0.5 g saturated fat), 7 g of protein, 510 mg of sodium, 41 g of carb, 5 g of fiber

GRILLED BASIL CHICKEN AND ZUCCHINI

Ingredients:

- 1 cup of white rice
- 1 lime, and wedges for serving purposes
- 2 garlic cloves
- 1 tablespoon of low-sodium soy sauce
- Half teaspoon of sugar
- Half red chile, finely sliced
- 4 small-sized zucchini (about 1 1/4 lbs.), sliced lengthwise
- 2 tablespoon of olive oil,
- Kosher salt and pepper to add flavor
- 1 lb. of chicken tenders
- 2 and a half cup of basil, unevenly chopped

Preparation:

Start cooking rice as per the directions mentioned on the package.

Zest lime into the large-sized bowl, then squeeze in 2 tablespoons of juice. Lightly grate garlic into a bowl, then stir in sugar, soy sauce, and chile.

Coat zucchini with 1 tablespoon of oil and flavor with 1/4 teaspoon of each salt and pepper. Rub chicken tenders with remaining tablespoon of oil and flavor with 1/4 teaspoon of each salt and pepper. Grill zucchini until hardly tender and chicken until well-cooked, around 3 minutes per side; shift to board.

Cut chicken and zucchini into pieces and toss in sauce; fold in basil and serve over rice with lime wedges.

Nutrition per serving: 400 calories in total, 10.5 g of fat (1.5 g saturated), 29 g of protein, 450 mg of sodium, 46 g of carb, 3 g of fiber

CHICAGO-STYLE CHICKEN DOGS

Ingredients:

- 2 jarred-pepperoncini peppers, finely sliced, also 1 tablespoon of brine
- 1 teaspoon of honey
- 1 teaspoon of yellow mustard, even more for serving
- 1 teaspoon of poppy seeds
- 1/4 small-sized sweet onion, finely sliced
- 4 well-cooked chicken sausages
- 4 hot dog buns
- 2 small-sized plum tomatoes, cubed into half-moons
- 4 dill pickle spears
- 1 small-sized romaine heart, finely sliced (around 3 cups)

Preparation:

Start heating the grill on medium heat. In a bowl, beat together pepperoncini brine, honey, and mustard; blend in poppy seeds. Add onion and pepperoncini peppers and toss to coat.

Now Grill sausages, turning rarely, until lightly overdone and heated through, about 10 to 12 minutes. If wished, grill buns.

Stuff sausages into buns alongside with tomatoes and pickles. Toss onions and poppy seeds with romaine and spoon sausages on top. Serve with remaining romaine mixture and extra mustard if needed.

Nutrition per serving: 490 calories in total, 16 g of fat (3 g saturated), 18 g of protein, 520 mg of sodium, 66 g of carb, 6 g of fiber

STEAK AND RYE PANZANELLA

Ingredients:

- 2 teaspoons of caraway seeds
- 2 tablespoon of red wine vinegar
- 4 tablespoon of olive oil, divided
- 1 tablespoon of whole-grain mustard
- 1 garlic clove, crushed
- Kosher salt and pepper to add flavor
- 1 bulb fennel, divided
- 1 medium-sized red onion, sliced into rounds
- 3 slices of rye bread (1 inch thick)
- 1 large of bunch kale, leaves minced (about 10 cups)
- 1 lb. of sirloin steak

Preparation:

Toast caraway seeds in a small pot on medium heat, around 2 minutes. In a small bowl, beat together vinegar, 2 tablespoons of oil, mustard, garlic, caraway seeds, and ¼ teaspoon of salt.

Start heat grill or grill pan on medium to high temperature. Coat fennel, onion, and bread with 1 tablespoon of oil and flavor fennel and onion with one pinch of salt. Grill, covered, frequently turning until vegetables are tender and overdone and bread is toasted, about 5 to 8 mins for vegetables and 1 to 2 mins for bread. Shift to cutting board; core and thinly slice fennel and tear bread into chunks.

In a large bowl, toss grilled vegetables, kale, and bread with half of the dressing and let sit, tossing infrequently.

Meanwhile, rub steak with the remaining 1 tablespoon of olive oil and flavor with ½ teaspoon of each salt and pepper. Grill as per your requirement, about 4 to 6 minutes per side for medium-rare. Shift to a cutting board and let it rest for about 5 minutes before slicing. Fold into the salad and sprinkle with remaining vinaigrette.

Nutrition per serving: 435 calories in total, 23 g of fat (5 g saturated), 29 g of protein, 735 mg of sodium, 28 g of carb, 6 g of fiber

Cheesy Tex-Mex Stuffed Chicken

Ingredients:

- 2 scallions (finely sliced)
- 2 seeded jalapeños (finely sliced)
- 1 1/4 cup of cilantro
- 1 teaspoon of lime zest
- 4 oz. of Monterey Jack cheese (coarsely grated)
- 4 small-sized of boneless, skinless chicken breasts
- 3 tablespoon of olive oil
- Salt and Pepper to add flavor
- 3 tablespoon of lime juice
- 2 bell peppers (finely cubed)
- Half small-sized red onion (finely sliced)
- 5 cup of torn romaine lettuce

Preparation:

Preheat the oven to a temperature of 450°F. In a bowl, mix scallions and seeded jalapeños, 1/4 cup of cilantro (minced) and lime zest, and toss with Monterey Jack cheese.

Put a knife into the thickest part of each of boneless, skinless chicken breasts and move back and forth to create 2 and 1/2-inch pocket that is as wide as possible without going through. Stuff chicken with a mixture of cheese

Heat 02 tablespoons of olive oil in a large pot on medium heat. Flavor chicken with salt and pepper and cook until it becomes brown on 1 side, about 3 to 4 minutes. Turn chicken pieces over and roast until well-cooked, about 10 to 12 minutes.

Meanwhile, in a large bowl, beat together lime juice, 1 tablespoon of olive oil and half teaspoon of salt. Now add bell peppers and red onion and let sit for about 10 minutes, tossing infrequently. Toss with romaine lettuce and 1 cup of fresh cilantro. Serve with chicken and lime wedges.

Nutrition per serving: 360 calories in total, 22 g of fat (7.5 g saturated), 32 g of protein, 715 mg of sodium, 10 g of carb, 3 g of fiber

Chapter 05: Appetizing Snacks For Weight Loss

Avocado Fries with Lime Dipping Sauce

Ingredients

- 8 ounces of small avocados (02), skinned, pitted and cut into 16 slices

- Large egg, slightly beaten (01)

- 3/4 cup of panko breadcrumbs, Gluten-Free can also be used

- 1 & 1/4 teaspoons of lime chili seasoning salt, like Tajin Classic

- For the lime dipping sauce:

- 1/4 cup of 0% Greek Yogurt

- 3 tablespoons of light mayonnaise

- 2 teaspoons of fresh lime juice

- 1/2 teaspoon of lime chili seasoning salt, like Tajin Classic

- 1/8 teaspoon of kosher salt

Preparation:

Air Fryer Directions:

Preheat the air-fryer at a temperature of 390F degrees.

Place egg in a shallow container. On a separate plate, mix panko with 1 teaspoon of Tajin.

Flavor avocado wedges with 1/4 teaspoon of Tajin. Dip each piece in egg first, and then in panko.

Sprinkle both sides with oil, then move to the air fryer and cook for about 7 to 8 minutes turning halfway. Serve hot with dipping sauce.

Oven Directions:

Preheat the oven 425F, follow directions above, and bake on a sheet pan until golden and crisp, 10 to 15 minutes.

Nutrition Per Serving:

"Calories: 197kcal, Carbohydrates: 15g, Protein: 7g, Fat: 12.5 g, saturated fat: 2g: Cholesterol: 94 mg, Sodium: 520 mg: Fiber: 4g. Sugar: 1.5g

Mango-Raspberry Fruit Roll-ups

Ingredients

- 1 large-sized ripped mango, skinned and sliced
- 6 ounces of fresh raspberries
- 2 tablespoons of sugar

Preparation:

Preheat the oven to a temperature of 150°F. Place a rimmed 12½ by 17¼-inch (half- sheet pan with a silicone baking mat.

In a mixer, mix the mango until its smooth. Now shift the mango to a bowl and place it aside. Add the raspberries and sugar to the mixer and blend until its smooth. (It is essential to blend the raspberries with the sugar, as the sugar helps to liquefy the berries.)

Put dollops of the mango and raspberry purées on the prepared pan. With the help of small offset spatula, spread the mashes evenly over the pantry to evenly spread them, not too thick and not too thin, and also not to spread them to the very ends, so you will have more space to grab the fruit leather and peel it off the rug when it's cool.

Bake for about 2 hours 30 minutes to 3 hours, spinning the baking sheet every hour. The leather is done when it is still viscous but not too sticky or wet. Let it cool.

Remove it from the rug and place it on top of a sheet with wax paper. Cut the leather and wax paper into strips with cutters and roll them up paper-side out, then store them in a sealed container at room temperature up to a week.

Nutrition Per Serving: "Calories: 39kcal, Carbohydrates: 10g, Cholesterol: 10mg, Sodium: 0.5mg, Fiber: 2g, Sugar: 7.5g"

DOUBLE CHOCOLATE PALEO BANANA BREAD

Ingredients

- 3 medium-sized overripe bananas (ones with brown spots are best)
- Large eggs 02
- 1 teaspoon of vanilla extract
- 3/4 cup of packed blanched fine almond flour
- 1/3 cup of packed coconut flour
- Half cup of high-quality cocoa powder (see recipe notes below)
- Half teaspoon of baking soda
- Half teaspoon of baking powder
- Half teaspoon of salt
- Half cup of chocolate chips, dairy-free if wished

For the additional topping:

- 2 tablespoons of chocolate chips (dairy-free, if wished)

- 1 teaspoon of coconut oil

Preparation:

Preheat oven to a temperature of 350 degrees Sprinkle an 8x8 inch baking pan with nonstick cooking spray and place it aside.

Add eggs, banana, and vanilla to a mixture and mix until the mixture is smooth.

Take a large bowl, beat together coconut flour, almond flour, cocoa powder, baking powder, baking soda, and salt.

Gradually fold in the wet mixture and stir until mixed well. Now stir in chocolate chunks, reserving a few tablespoons.

Spread the batter equally into the prepared pot and spray remaining chocolate chunks on top. Bake for about 18-25 minutes or until the toothpick comes out clean. Once baking is done, shift pan to a wire rack to cool for about 20 minutes before slicing into 12 bars.

Nutrition Per Serving:

Servings: 12 bars Serving size: 1 bar Calories: 159kcal Fat: 9.1g Carbohydrates: 15.5g Fiber: 4.2g Sugar: 6.4g Protein: 3g

Air Fryer Tostones (Twice Air-Fried Plantains)

Ingredients

- 1 large-sized green plantain, ends clipped and skinned "6 oz "
- Olive Oil to sprinkle
- 1 cup of water
- 1 teaspoon of kosher salt
- 3/4 teaspoon of garlic powder

Preparation:

With the help of a sharp knife and cut a slit along the length of the plantain skin, it will make it stress-free to peel. Cut the plantain into inch pieces and cut 8 pieces in total.

Take a small bowl and mix the water with salt and garlic powder.

Preheat the air fryer up to a temperature of 400F.

When it's ready, sprinkle the plantain with olive oil and cook for about 6 minutes, this might be completed in two batches

Now take it from the air fryer and while they are hot purée them with a tostonera or the bottom of a jar or measuring cup to crush or to flatten

Dip them in the flavored water and place it aside.

Preheat the air fryer to the temperature of 400F once again and start cooking in batches, five mins on each side, sprinkle both sides of the plantains with olive oil.

When it's done, give them another spritz of oil and flavor with salt. Enjoy it!

Nutrition Per Serving:

4tostones, Calories: 102kcal, Carbohydrates: 27g, Protein: 1g, Sodium: 250mg, Fiber: 2g, Sugar: 12g

Delicious Carrot Cake Cookies (Prepared with Coconut Oil & Dairy-Free!

Ingredients

- 3/4 cup of white whole wheat flour
- Half teaspoon of baking soda
- 1/4 teaspoon of salt
- 1 & 1/2 teaspoons of cinnamon
- 1/8 teaspoon of nutmeg
- 1/4 cup of coconut oil, melted and cooled
- 1/2 cup of packed dark brown sugar (or sub coconut sugar)
- 1 medium-sized egg
- 1 teaspoon of vanilla extract
- 1 heaping cup of shredded carrots
- 1 1/4 cups of rolled oats

- 1/3 cup of unsweetened shredded coconut
- 1/4 cup of chopped pecans or walnuts
- 1/4 cup of raisins

For the coating:

- 1/4 cup of powdered sugar
- 1-2 teaspoons of unsweetened almond milk
- Sprint of cinnamon

Preparation:

Preheat oven to a temperature of 350 degrees F. Place a baking sheet with parchment paper.

Take a medium-sized bowl, beat together baking soda, flour, cinnamon, nutmeg, and salt.

Take a large-sized separate bowl and combine brown sugar, coconut oil, egg, and vanilla until well mixed; then fold in shredded carrots. Add in flour mixture and blend with a wooden spoon until just mixed. Fold in pecans, oats, coconut, and raisins.

Take a small cookie scoop and drop by tablespoonful on a baking sheet. Smoothly flatten with your hand. Bake for about 9-11 minutes or until it changes color around the corners. Cool cookies for about a few minutes on the baking sheet before shifting to a wire rack to finish cooling.

For the glaze: Mix powdered sugar, almond milk, and cinnamon in a medium-sized bowl. Sprinkle a tiny bit over cookies, then let dry. Makes around 18 cookies.

Nutrition Per Servings: 18 cookies Serving size: 1 cookie Calories: 136kcal Fat: 6.6g Carbohydrates: 18.1g Fiber: 2g Sugar: 9g Protein: 2.4g

No-Bake Superfood Brownie Energy Bars

Ingredients:

For the bars:

- 1 cup of packed pitted Medjool dates
- 1/4 cup of raw walnuts
- 1/4 cup of raw pecans halves
- Half cup of shelled pistachios, divided
- 1/4 cup of unsweetened shredded coconut
- 1 tablespoon of chia seeds
- 3 tablespoons of unsweetened cocoa powder (or cacao powder)
- 1 tablespoon of melted virgin coconut oil
- 1 teaspoon of vanilla
- 1/4 teaspoon of sea salt
- 1/4 cup of goji berries or cherries (dried)

- 1 tablespoon of warm water, if required

For the topping

- 1.5 ounces of 85% dark chocolate (vegan, if wished)

For Garnishing:

- 1 tablespoon of shelled pistachios
- 1 tablespoon of goji berries
- 1 tablespoon of chopped pecans
- Maldon sea salt, for drizzling on top

Preparation:

Add only ¼ cup of pistachios, dates, walnuts, pecans to the bowl of a food mixture. Process until its chunky.

Now add in chia seeds, cocoa powder, unsweetened shredded coconut, coconut oil, and vanilla extract. Start again until the mixture is chunky and marginally clumping. If the combination is dry, add 1-2 tablespoons of warm water in it.

Now add the remaining ¼ cup of pistachios and goji berries and mix a few times again until pistachios are somewhat chunky. Add this mixture into an 8x4 inch loaf pot lined with parchment paper, pressing equally towards the sides of the pan.

Add dark chocolate to a small pot and place it on low heat until it melts. You can use the microwave with 30-second increments, stirring in between until chocolate is fully liquefied and smooth.

Drizzle over the bars, tilting pot so that the chocolate covers the bars equally. Relish the bars with 1 tablespoon of these ingredients: goji berries, pistachios, and crushed pecans.

Put these bars in the freezer for about 30 minutes-1 hour to solidify. Once it's ready to serve, drizzle with Maldon sea salt and cut into 8 pieces. Store in the freezer (covered) for up to 1 month. Enjoy!

ature*Nutrition Per Serving*: 8 squares Serving Size: 1 bar Calories: 234kcal Fat: 14.2g Carbohydrates: 26.9g Fiber: 6g Sugar: 18.2g Protein: 4.5g

Homemade Chunky Healthy Granola Recipe (Vegan & Gluten-Free!)

Ingredients:

Dry ingredients:

- 2 cups of old fashioned rolled oats, gluten-free

- Half cup oat flour, gluten-free if wished

- 2 tablespoons of flaxseed meal
- 2 tablespoons of white sesame seeds
- 3/4 cup of sliced raw almonds
- 3/4 cup of raw pecans halves
- 3/4 cup of raw cashews
- 2 teaspoons of ground cinnamon
- Half teaspoon of sea salt
- Wet ingredients:

- 1/4 cup of coconut oil

- 1/3 cup of pure maple syrup

- 1 teaspoon of vanilla extract

- Half cup packed of pitted Medjool dates, crushed

- Half cup of golden raisins

Preparation

Preheat oven to a temperature of 300 degrees F. Line a large-sized baking sheet with parchment paper.

Take a large-sized bowl, beat together oats, sesame seeds, almonds, oat flour, flaxseed meal, pecans, cashews cinnamon, and salt.

Now add maple syrup, coconut oil, and vanilla extract to a small pot and place it on low heat, stirring regularly until coconut oil is completely liquefied. Pour all the dry ingredients and mix well until oats are completely covered.

Next, spread the granola equally in the baking pan and bake for about 20 minutes.

After 20 minutes' stir granola and bake for around 15-20 minutes longer or until granola just slightly changes color. Remove from the oven and allow it to cool completely on the baking sheet, so that little clumps stay together.

Once it's cooled, stir in crushed dates and raisins. Shift to a sealed container or large mason jar. Best used within 7 to 10 days.

Nutrition Per Serving:

Servings: 18 servings Serving size: 0.25 cup Calories: 210kcal Fat: 12.3g Saturated fat: 3.8g Carbohydrates: 22.9g Fiber: 3.4g Sugar: 10.5g Protein: 4.1g

Vegetarian Plantain & Black Bean Taco Cups

Ingredients

- 1 package of "8-inch" flour tortillas
- Half tablespoon of olive oil or avocado oil
- 2 cloves garlic, crushed
- Half cup of cubed white onion
- 1 slightly underripe plantain, cubed
- 1 jalapeno, seeded and cubed
- Salt and pepper
- 1 cup of Black Beans in a Mild Chili Sauce,
- 3 ounces of manchego cheese, shredded (about ¾ cup)

For serving:

- 1-2 ripe avocados, Depending on your requirement
- Freshly ground salt and pepper, to enhance test
- Freshly squeezed lime juice, from half small-sized lime

- Freshly chopped cilantro

Preparation:

Preheat oven to a temperature of 350 degrees F. Lubricates a 12 cup muffin pan with olive oil cooking spray.

Using a biscuit cutter to cut out 3 ½- 4-inch pieces from your tortillas. Place round tortilla slices in each muffin liner.

Add olive oil to a medium-sized pan and place it on medium to high temperature. Add in crushed garlic, cubed plantains, and cubed jalapeno—flavor with salt and pepper. Cook for about 5-8 minutes until onion is tender.

Remove from heat and stir in Chili Beans. Spread the plantain chili bean mixture equally between tortilla cups.

Bake for about 10-15 minutes, then remove and drizzle shredded cheese on top. Bake for about 3-5 minutes so that cheese melts.

While taco cups are baking, mash 1 ripe avocado in a medium-sized bowl—flavor with salt and pepper and a little fresh lime juice. Mash everything together until mixed well.

Top each taco cup with crushed avocado and a drizzle of cilantro. Add a little hot sauce on top if you want!

Nutrition Per Servings: 12 servings Serving size: 1 taco cup Calories: 134kcal Fat: 5.4g Saturated fat: 1.6g Carbohydrates: 17.6g Fiber: 2.6g Sugar: 2.3g Protein: 4.4g

GREEN GODDESS HUMMUS

Ingredients:

- 1/4 cup of tahini

- 1/4 cup of fresh lemon juice (1 large Lemon)

- 2 tablespoons of olive oil, plus more for serving the purpose

- Half cup of roughly chopped, fresh parsley (loosely packed)

- 1/4 cup of roughly chopped, fresh tarragon (loosely packed)

- 2 to 3 tablespoons of roughly chopped fresh chives or green onion

- 1 large garlic clove, roughly crushed

- Half teaspoon of salt, more to enhance taste

- 01 "15-ounce" can of chickpeas, rinsed and drained

- 1 to 2 tablespoons of water, optional

- Decorate with extra olive oil and a drizzle of chopped fresh herbs

Preparation:

Mix the tahini and lemon juice in the bowl of your food mixer. Mix for about 1 and a half minutes, pausing to fix down the bowl of your mixture as necessary.

Add the tarragon, chives, olive oil, parsley, crushed garlic, and salt to the beaten tahini and lemon juice mixture. Mix for about 1 minute, pausing to fix down the bowl as essential.

Add half of the chickpeas to the food mixture and mixture for 1 minute. Scrape down the container, then add the remaining chickpeas and mix for until the hummus is thick and quite smooth, around 1 to 2 minutes more.

If the hummus is too thick or hasn't yet mixed into creamy oblivion, run the food mixture while sprinkling in 1 to 2 tablespoons of water until it matches your desired consistency.

Scrape the hummus into a small-sized serving bowl. Sprinkle about a tablespoon of olive oil on top and drizzle with additional chopped herbs.

Store hummus in a sealed container and refrigerate for up to 1 week.

Nutrition Per serving: 142 calories, 9.6 g fat, 11.6 g carbs, 3 g fiber, 4.5 g protein

CRISPY BAKED SWEET POTATO FRIES

Ingredients

- 2 pounds of sweet potatoes (about 2 medium to large-sized)
- 1 tablespoon of cornstarch
- Half teaspoon of fine sea salt
- 2 tablespoons of extra-virgin olive oil
- freshly ground black pepper, cayenne pepper or garlic powder (to enhance the taste)

Preparation

Preheat the oven to a temperature of 425 degrees Fahrenheit with racks in the lower and upper thirds of the oven. Line two large-sized, rimmed baking sheets with parchment paper as it allows the fries not to stuck to the pans.

Skin the sweet potatoes and cut them into fry-shaped pieces. Try to cut them into similarly sized pieces so the fries will bake equally. Shift half of the uncooked fries to one baking sheet and the other half to another baking sheet.

Drizzle the sweet potato fries with the cornstarch and salt. Mix until the fries are slightly covered in powder. Sprinkle the olive oil over the fries (1 tablespoon per pan) and mix until the fries are slightly and equally covered in oil, and no powdery spots remain

Place your fries in a single layer and don't overcrowd them; otherwise, they will not crisp up. Bake for about 20 minutes, then flip the fries so they can be cooked from all sides.

Position the fries in even layers across the saucepan again, moving any browned fries more toward the middle of the pan so they won't get overcooked. Return the saucepans to the oven, swap their positions.

Bake for about 10 to 18 additional minutes, or until the fries are crunchy. You'll know they're almost done when the surface of the fries changes from shiny orange to a more matte, puffed up texture. Sometimes the lower pan will be done a few minutes before the top pan. Don't worry if the corners are a little bit brown; they will taste more caramelized than burnt.

If wished, toss the baked fries with different flavors to enhance the taste. Serve warm!

Nutrition Per serving: 263 calories, 7.1 g fat, 47.4 g carbs, 6.8 g fiber, 3.6 g protein

CREAMY PEACH & HONEY POPSICLES

Ingredients

- 1 pound of ripe peaches (medium-sized), skinned and cubed into ½-inch wide wedges

- 6 tablespoons of honey, divided

- Pinch of sea salt

- 2 cups of full fat/whole milk plain yogurt (regular or Greek)

- 1 tablespoon of lemon juice (1 lemon small-sized, juiced)

- Half teaspoon of vanilla extract

Preparation:

Preheat oven to a temperature of 350 degrees Fahrenheit. Line a rimmed baking sheet with parchment paper. Shift cubed peaches to the baking sheet and lightly toss with 2 tablespoons of honey and a pinch of salt. Position the peaches in a single layer. Roast for around 30 - 40 minutes, stirring halfway, or until the peaches are juicy and soft.

While the fruit is roasting, mix the yogurt, ¼ cup of honey, lemon juice, and vanilla extract in a medium-sized bowl. Feel free to add extra honey or vanilla extract to suit your taste buds. Place the blend in the refrigerator, so it stays cool.

Allow the peaches to cool, then scrape the peaches and all of their juices into the bowl of yogurt. Use a big-sized spoon to fold the mixture together slightly.

Use the spoon to shift the yogurt blend into the popsicle mould. You may have to push the peaches down into the molds, but they shouldn't put up too much of a fight. Insert popsicle sticks and freeze for around four hours.

When it's ready to pop out the popsicles, run warm water around the outsides of the moulds for around ten seconds, and slightly remove the popsicles. Enjoy the meal.

Nutrition Per serving (1 popsicle): 170 calories, 4.4 g fat, 31.3 g carbs, 1.3 g fiber, 3.9 g protein

Protein Cookie Dough

Ingredients

- 1 "15 oz" can of chickpeas, rinsed.
- 1/4 cup of vanilla vegan protein powder
- 2 Tablespoons of almond butter or cashew butter
- 1 Tablespoon of coconut sugar
- 1 teaspoon of vanilla extract
- 1/8 teaspoon of sea salt
- 2 Tablespoons of dairy-free chocolate chips

Preparation

Add chickpeas to a large food mixer and mix until they start to smooth out. You might need to use a rubber spatula to scrape down the corners.

Add the remaining ingredients, including protein powder, vanilla, nut butter, coconut sugar, sea salt, and mix until a ball of dough forms.

Using a rubber spatula, separate the dough a bit, add chocolate chips, and beat 2-3 times or until chocolate chips get distributed in the dough.

Remove dough from the mixer, and enjoy it!

For a cookie dough sundae with the chocolate sprinkle: simply use an ice cream scoop to scoop the dough into a small-sized bowl. Melt 1-2 Tablespoons additional chocolate chips with a half teaspoon of coconut oil in the microwave for about 15-20 seconds and Sprinkle over the cookie dough. Enjoy.

For cookie dough balls: roll the dough by using a heaping Tablespoon into balls. These can also be soaked in chocolate for chocolate coated cookie dough bites.

For cookie dough dip: add almond milk (about 1/4 or so) for a thinner touch that's perfect for soaking. Serve with apple slices or graham crackers.

Store remaining dough in the fridge for up to 3 to 4 days.

Nutrition Per serving (¼ cup): 164 calories, 5 g fat, 19 g carbs, 4 g fiber, 10 g protein

Almond Joy Protein Balls

Ingredients

- One and a half cups of old-fashioned rolled oats
- 1 cup natural of almond butter
- 1/4 cup of honey
- 2 scoops "64 grams" of chocolate protein powder
- 1–2 Tablespoons of unsweetened shredded coconut

Preparation

Place honey, protein powder oats, almond butter, and shredded coconut in a large bowl and stir to combine.

Getting the mixture to mix takes a little arm muscle, and it may seem too thick in the beginning, but it will come together as you keep blending.

Once it's mixed, use a small cookie scoop to scoop and form the dough into balls.

Store in a sealed container in the fridge

Nutrition Per serving (1 ball): 109 calories, 7 g fat, 9 g carbs, 2 g fiber, 5 g protein

BAKED KALE CHIPS

Ingredients

- 1 bunch of curly kale (about 5 cups)
- 1 Tablespoon of olive oil
- Half teaspoon of sea salt

Preparation

Preheat oven to a temperature of 350°F.

Rinse and dry kale, de-stem and roughly slice into bite-size pieces.

Make sure kale is completely dry, add to a large-sized bowl, and mix with olive oil and sea salt.

Distribute kale out on a large-sized baking sheet, ensuring not to overlap pieces.

Bake for about 15-20 minutes, until kale is crispy.

Best served instantly, but if wished, you can also store them in a sealed container for about 1 to 2 days.

Nutrition Per serving (1 bunch): 184 calories, 14 g fat, 7 g carbs, 3 g fiber, 3 g protein

Chocolate Covered Banana Pops

Ingredients

- 4 medium-sized bananas
- 6 "oz" of chocolate chips
- One and a half tablespoons of coconut oil
- 3 Tablespoons of chopped almonds and shredded coconut
- Bamboo skewers or popsicle sticks (08)

Preparation

Line a small baking sheet with parchment paper.

Skin each banana. Remove peels and cut each banana in half.

Add a bamboo skewer or popsicle stick into each banana half.

Lay bananas on a baking sheet and freeze for about 1 hour or until bananas are freezing.

Melt the coconut oil and chocolate together. Microwave can also be used for this. In a microwave, add chocolate and coconut oil into a safe bowl. Heat it for about a minute, stir and continue to heat with 30-second increments until chocolate is entirely melted and smooth.

Dip freezing banana half into the melted chocolate, cover as much of the banana as you would like. Drizzle with almonds or coconut to garnish. Do the procedure quickly before chocolate hardens

Position chocolate-coated banana back on the parchment-lined baking sheet and repeat this process until all the bananas are covered. Enjoy immediately or store any remaining banana pops in the refrigerator for up to a month.

Nutrition Per serving (1 pop): 144 calories, 9 g fat, 21 g carbs, 6 g fiber, 2 g protein

Vitamin C Boosting Tropical Green Smoothie

Ingredients

- 1 cup of dark baby greens spinach, kale
- Half cup of pineapple chunks
- Half cup of mango chunks
- Kiwi (01)
- 1 tablespoon of chia seeds reserve some for decoration if wished
- 2 tablespoons of rolled oats (optional)
- Half cup of water
- Half cup of ice
- 1 teaspoon of coconut flakes

Preparation

Mix all ingredients except coconut flakes in a high-speed mixture and blend until smooth. Relish with coconut flakes and reserved chia seeds, if wished.

Nutrition Per Serving: Calories 283, Total Fat: 7.1g 1   1   %
Cholesterol 0g 0%, Sodium: 30.4mg 1%, Total Carbohydrate 53g, 18% Dietary Fiber: 11.7g, 47% Sugars: 25.9g

FRUIT SALAD WITH CITRUS-MINT DRESSING

For the Dressing

Ingredients

- 1 tablespoon of honey
- Juice of half a lime
- Juice of half a lemon
- 1 tablespoon of minced mint, plus extra for decoration

For the Salad

- 1 cup of blueberries
- 1 cup of quartered strawberries
- 6 ounces of blackberries
- 1 large-sized banana, skinned and sliced

Preparation:

Mix all the ingredients for the dressing in a small-sized bowl.

Place all the fruit in a large-sized bowl. Pour the dressing on the top and toss to cover the fruit. Decorate with more fresh mint and serve.

Nutrition Per serving (¼ of recipe): 117 calories, 0.8 g fat, 28.8 g carbs, 5 g fiber, 1.7 g protein

Conclusion

Weight Loss is an essential part of weight management. It is imperative because being overweight is not good for your health. Weighing too much increases your risk of health conditions like heart problems, type 2 diabetes, high blood pressure, and most prominently cancer. Excessive weight can also increase your risk for sleep apnea (abnormal breathing at night), osteoarthritis (joint disease), and other respiratory problems. Also, it may also cause an individual to feel sad or be treated differently by other people

The perfect way to lose weight is by consuming fewer calories (the energy units that your body gets from food) and exercising daily. Consuming more calories than you need will become a reason for you to gain weight. Try to reduce your calories by 500 calories per day. Undoubtedly, this book will provide you with a number of recipes to help you lose weight. Along with the meal recipes, you can also burn calories if you exercise daily. You will certainly experience a significant difference in your health. Also, you will feel improved physical health as well as energy levels.

Final Words

Thank you again for purchasing this book!

We hope this book can help you.

The next step is for you to **join our email newsletter** to receive updates on any upcoming new book releases or promotions. You can sign-up for free, and as a bonus, you will also receive our "*7 Fitness Mistakes You Don't Know You're Making*" book! This bonus book breaks down many of the most common fitness mistakes and will demystify many of the complexities and science of getting into shape. Having all this fitness knowledge and science organized into an actionable step-by-step book will help you get started in the right direction in your fitness journey! To join our free email newsletter and grab your free book, please visit the link and signup: **www.effingopublishing.com/gift**

Finally, if you enjoyed this book, then we would like to ask you for a favor, would you be kind enough to leave a review for this book? It would be greatly appreciated! Thank you, and good luck on your journey!

ABOUT THE CO-AUTHORS

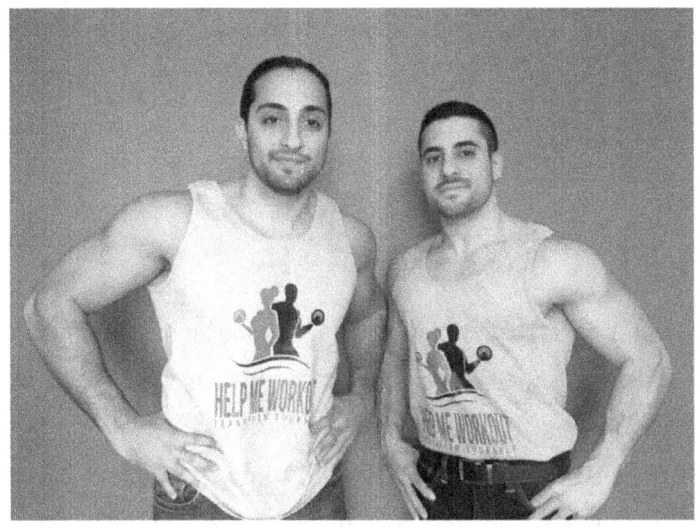

Our name is Alex & George Kaplo; we're both certified personal trainers from Montreal, Canada. We will start by saying we are not the biggest guys you will ever meet, and this has never really been our goal. We started working out to overcome our biggest insecurity when we were younger, which was our self-confidence. You may be going through some challenges right now, or you may simply want to get fit, and we can certainly relate.

We always kind were interested in the health & fitness world and wanted to gain some muscle due to the numerous bullying in our teenage years. We figured we could do something about how our body looks like. This was the beginning of our transformation journey. We had no idea where to start, but we both just got started. We felt worried and afraid at times that other people would make fun of us for doing the exercises the wrong way. We always wished we had a friend to guide us and who could just show us the ropes.

After a lot of work, studying, and countless trials and errors. Some people began to notice how we were both getting more fit and how we were starting to form a keen interest in the topic. This led many friends and new faces to come to us and ask us for fitness advice. At first, it seemed odd when people asked us to help them get in shape. But what kept us going is when they started to see changes in their own body and told us it's the first time that they saw real results! From there, more people kept coming to us, and it made both of us realize after so much reading and studying in this field that it did help us, but it also allowed us to help others. To date, we have coached and trained numerous clients who have achieved some pretty amazing results.

Today, both of us own & operate this publishing business, where we bring passionate and expert authors to write about health and fitness topics. We also run an online fitness business, and we would love to connect with you by inviting you to visit the website on the following page and signing up for our e-mail newsletter (you will even get a free book).

Last but not least, if you are in the position we were once in and you want some guidance, don't hesitate and ask... We will be there to help you out!

Your coaches,

Alex & George Kaplo

Download another book for Free

We want to thank you for purchasing this book and offer you another book (just as long and valuable as this book), "Health & Fitness Mistakes You Don't Know You're Making," completely free.

Visit the link below to signup and receive it:

www.effingopublishing.com/gift

In this book, we will break down the most common health & fitness mistakes, you are probably committing right now, and will reveal how you can easily get in the best shape of your life!

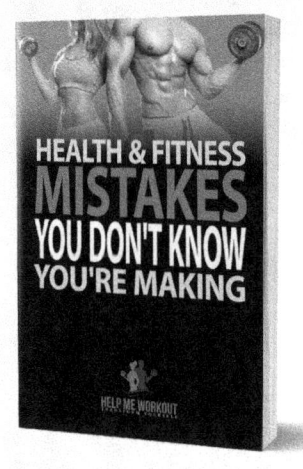

In addition to this valuable gift, you will also have an opportunity to get our new books for free, enter giveaways, and receive other valuable emails from us. Again, visit the link to sign up:

www.effingopublishing.com/gift

Copyright 2019 by Effingo Publishing - All Rights Reserved.

This document by Effingo Publishing, owned by the A&G Direct Inc company, is geared towards providing exact and reliable information in regards to the topic and issue covered. The publication is sold with the idea that the publisher is not required to render accounting, officially permitted or otherwise qualified services. If advice is necessary, legal or professional, a practiced individual in the profession should be ordered.

From a Declaration of Principles, which was accepted and approved equally by a Committee of the American Bar Association and a Committee of Publishers and Associations.

In no way is it legal to reproduce, duplicate, or transmit any part of this document in either electronic means or printed format. Recording of this publication is strictly prohibited, and any storage of this document is not allowed unless with written permission from the publisher. All rights reserved.

The information provided herein is stated to be truthful and consistent, in that any liability, in terms of inattention or otherwise, by any usage or abuse of any policies, processes, or directions contained within is the solitary and utter responsibility of the recipient reader. Under no circumstances will any legal responsibility or blame be held against the publisher for any reparation, damages, or monetary loss due to the information herein, either directly or indirectly.

The information herein is offered for informational purposes solely and is universal as so. The presentation of the information is without a contract or any type of guarantee assurance.

The trademarks that are used are without any consent, and the publication of the trademark is without permission or backing by the trademark owner. All trademarks and brands within this book are for clarifying purposes only and are owned by the owners themselves, not affiliated with this document.

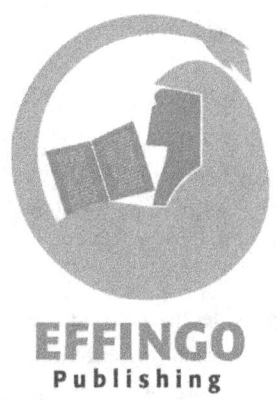

For more great books, visit:

EffingoPublishing.com

www.ingramcontent.com/pod-product-compliance
Lightning Source LLC
Chambersburg PA
CBHW070903080526
44589CB00013B/1164